The

Motivator

Guide to

Abs

A brief overview of the writer:

Kurt Motivator is a fitness and nutrition fanatic, with over a decade of experience in fitness and weight training combined. As a young boy Kurt Motivator had an unwavering interest in sports and specifically athletics and football. As he grew into adolescence he continued his passion and went on to play for Wolverhampton Wanderers youth for a number of years before suffering a serious hip injury (Slipped Upper Femoral Epithasis) and being told that he would certainly never continue along the path of a football career again; but even more disturbingly... That he could potentially "Never Walk Again". After numerous operations and sometimes spending 12 weeks+ at a time in hospital beds; Kurt decided to take a different path in life. At this point he took up Information Technology as a new hobby, interest and career path and decided to focus all of his energy in this area. Fast forward a couple of years and Kurt had developed the habits of eating the wrong things; hardly exercising and generally not taking care of his physical appearance. A once super fit, energetic and aspiring professional footballer; now weighed in excess of 21 stones in weight, with huge amounts of body fat and internal fats (visceral fats). It was time to change. 2 1/2 years prior to this guide being written; Kurt decided that enough was enough, he dramatically changed his nutrition, training and lifestyle, lost in excess of 7 stone in body fat and now stands at 6ft 3inches at 14stone 6lb lean! Kurt is now a leader in the industry of wellbeing, he eats sleeps and lives an overall healthy lifestyle, is a public figure in the field of Nutrition and Motivation and has changed thousands of lives all around the planet. So, here we have it, some of Kurt Motivators best kept training secrets revealed! This is The Motivator Guide to Abs!

Welcome and *Congratulations* on your purchase of The Motivator Guide to Abdominals.

In this guide; I myself... Kurt Motivator will talk you through exactly how to achieve those wash board abs to make sure you are Spring, Summer, Autumn and Winter ready, who said that abs can only come around in the Summer?

First of all, I would like to open this guide by explaining something that so many people do not fully understand. In order to achieve great muscular definition, Lean Gains and those beach bodies; it's also imperative that we take care of our nutrition. In fact; it's so important that I can actually sit here today and tell you that to achieve fantastic physical results; it's actually 80% down to what you put into your mouth (don't be rude) and 20% Physical exercise. Anyway, if you would like to find out a little more on this topic, then I cover this in more detail in my guide "The Motivator Meal Plan" but for now we are talking Abs!

Before we get physical! I would like us to take a couple of moments to explore your thoughts. You're probably thinking; "aye? i purchased this guide to learn a few exercise tips" but it's important that we explore the way we currently see ourselves in order to create a new, improved mental picture with those abdominals you desire! So, at this point I would like you to take a moment, go into your mental bank of thoughts and think about 5 words that you would currently use to describe your "stomach, belly, emotional centre, core, gut" or whatever word you generally use to describe your middle region! How would you describe it? What do you see or say to yourself mentally when you look in the mirror?

Ok, so... You have probably realised at this point, that one of two things would have happened; 1) You are currently describing this area of your body a little negatively/ It doesn't give you the best of feelings to even think about looking at this area in the mirror. 2) You were super positive, felt great and stand in the mirror for most of the day taking mirror shots? (Cool Selfies)... In which case you either don't need the information I'm about to describe in this guide. Or you know exactly how to put forward positive images to attract the type of results you desire?

For a moment i would like to speak about the later. I would like to speak about creating your dream body and abs in your mind before we even go into our exercise regime. OK, you're going to have to trust me now? Is that ok... Good. What I would like you to do is picture in your mind exactly how it would feel to have your perfect set of abs. How would you act? What would you wear? How would you appear on the beach? How would your confidence change? Now really picture this. And now, i would like you to take a magazine/newspaper/go online and find a picture of a person who has the set of abdominals that you desire! You are going to need to put this image somewhere where you can see it each day (a secret place if you like, so people don't start to think you're strange). Now, the next step is; each and every time you see this picture; I would like you to say "Thank You for my Perfect Set of Abs". Now this is important; most people fall at the first hurdle by holding such a bad self-image of themselves and having so little self-belief that they can massively slow down their own results and commitment to this guide unless they are ready to change their mind-set! Give it a try!

Now it's time to get Physical! As always, I would suggest it's always a good idea to check with your doctor or physician before carrying out any of the exercises to follow; especially if you have any specific or major injuries. I am going to split the workout categories into 3 different levels, beginners, intermediate and advanced; this is for you to decide. I would suggest that everyone begins by testing out the beginner programme first of all, feel your way into the exercises, make sure you are not over doing it the first time and then increase the level accordingly. Oh and by the way, I have also added a FREE image guide that can be found in the final pages of this book to help you with your form and posture on each exercise!

The Motivator Workout

OK, so today is day 1! Once again I would like to congratulate you on taking this great step in the right direction! By now your mind should hold a new positive self-image and you are ready to "Rock and Roll". Now, of course I haven't bought you here today with your gym gear on and new sweat bang to just do those basic "Crunches" some of the exercises you will meet throughout this guide are the fundamentals to strong abs although I'm all about variation! Watch, learn and take part! (Each Day over the next 4 weeks will be dissected into 10 - 20 minute abdominal workouts aimed to "burn those biscuits" - It's important that you follow each day and do not take any days off. If you do miss a day/session it's important that you then go back 2 days, just go get back into the swing of things! No cheating!)

Disclaimer: It is very important that before you begin any exercise that you have completed a warm up and stretches accordingly. Kurt Motivator does not claim to be a doctor and physician and therefore advises that all individuals participating in "The Motivator Guide to Abs" should specifically warm up ad cool down prior to and after participating in any of the workouts to follow.

Day 1

Flutter Kicks

So here we are it's the first exercise of your new body! And today we are going to kick start our workout with some flutter kicks! This is a nice simple exercise to get started as i want to ease us into the next 4 weeks of activity and not frighten you off too soon! Ok, so first of all if you can get yourself into the neutral position, with your arms out by your side (or to make it a little bit easier you can place your hands underneath your bottom). Now, the next step is to raise both of your legs slightly so that they are a couple of inches off the ground (not too high). All you are going to do now is very small flutter kicks almost like you are swimming in shallow water and can only move your legs a little; but very quickly! Choose your ability level below; start your timer and let's hit it!

Beginner: 30 second burst of exercise for 3 sets (follow each set with a 30 second break)

Intermediate: 45 second burst of exercise for 3 sets (follow each set with a 30 second break)

Advanced: 1 minute burst of exercise for 3 sets (follow each set with a 30 second break)

Drunken Mountain Climbers

Yes you read it right! And it is definitely not the right time to be getting drunk. So for this exercise we are simply going to pretend! Many of you may be familiar with a basic mountain climber where from the neutral (high plank) position you will simply alternate and bring one knee at a time into your chest and then back to neutral! Well, the drunken mountain climber is very similar! However, this time we are going to bring our knee forward and across to the opposite elbow! That's right knee to left elbow, back to neutral and then left knee to right elbow! This little beauty is going to work our obliques, in simple terms; this is going to help us get rid of those love handles!

Beginner: 30 second burst of exercise for 3 sets (follow each set with a 30 second break)

Intermediate: 45 second burst of exercise for 3 sets (follow each set with a 30 second break)

Advanced: 1 minute burst of exercise for 3 sets (follow each set with a 30 second break)

Heel Touches

Now it's time to work those oblique's again with Heel Touches. Follow the example below; firstly going over towards one side, back to the centre (down) and then reaching over to the other side. It's important here that you keep the abs engaged throughout this exercise.

Beginner: 10 repetitions for 3 sets (30 second break between each set)

Intermediate: 15 repetitions for 3 sets (30 second break between each set)

Advanced: 20 repetitions for 3 sets (30 second break between each set)

Star Shape - Opposite Arm to Leg

Now it's time to make some snow angels (Just kidding). If you lie on the floor almost resembling a star with your arms and legs stretched out. All we are going to do here is raise the opposite arm to leg and meet in the middle. This is a great way to engage the abs and is personally one of my favourite. We are going to carry this exercise out for 3 sets, with a 30 second break between each set. Let's start!

Beginner: 10 repetitions for 3 sets (30 second break between each set)

Intermediate: 15 repetitions for 3 sets (30 second break between each set)

Advanced: 20 repetitions for 3 sets (30 second break between each set)

Cycling

So, here we have our final exercise for day 1! Who said training abs and getting healthy couldn't be fun too? In this exercise we are going to be cycling through the air with our Cycle Crunches! Don't worry if you are thinking... what on earth? Take a look at the image below which gives a great example of the perfect form for this exercise.

Beginner: 30 second burst of exercise for 3 sets (follow each set with a 30 second break)

Intermediate: 45 second burst of exercise for 3 sets (follow each set with a 30 second break)

Advanced: 1 minute burst of exercise for 3 sets (follow each set with a 30 second break)

Day 2

Reaching Oblique crunch

Welcome back! I hope you have had a good night's sleep because it's time to get to work for day 2! And we are going to start today's activities with some Oblique Crunches! Ok, so this one is pretty simple, all we are going to is crunch up and as we crunch, we are going to reach over to the outside of the opposite thigh. That means; right hand reaching over to the outside of the left thigh and vice versa! Let's go!

Beginner: 10 repetitions for 3 sets (30 second break between each set)

Intermediate: 15 repetitions for 3 sets (30 second break between each set)

Advanced: 20 repetitions for 3 sets (30 second break between each set)

Front leg raises

Good effort! Now it's lower abs time, who wants to lose that muffin top? Its time! What we are going to do here is elevate ourselves into the air using our arms and then alternatively raise each leg one at a time!

Beginner: 10 repetitions for 3 sets (30 second break between each set)

Intermediate: 15 repetitions for 3 sets (30 second break between each set)

Advanced: 20 repetitions for 3 sets (30 second break between each set)

Supermen or women

Superman or woman to the rescue! It's now time to stretch those abs out and work the core muscles! We are going to begin by lying flat with both our arms and legs stretched out! We are then simply going to stretch the core by raising both our arms and legs at the same time. (To the rescue) Don't worry, we all feel a little bit silly doing this one, but it's certainly relevant for those wash board abs.

Beginner: 10 repetitions for 3 sets (30 second break between each set)

Intermediate: 15 repetitions for 3 sets (30 second break between each set)

Advanced: 20 repetitions for 3 sets (30 second break between each set)

Plank (Raise Alternative Arms out in front)

Now, we're going to continue working our abs and core and begin to add some stability exercises to really increase your strength within this area! As shown in the image below, this exercise is going to start off looking like a raised plank, and all we are going to do is alternatively stretch our arms out in front! Please remember on this exercise that once both arms have been raised that is going to be 1 repetition! (As much as you would like it to be 1 repetition per arm!)

Beginner: 10 repetitions for 3 sets (30 second break between each set)

Intermediate: 15 repetitions for 3 sets (30 second break between each set)

Advanced: 20 repetitions for 3 sets (30 second break between each set)

Reverse crunches double leg

Time for our final exercise of Day 2! I am pretty much addicted to this exercise! If there is any one exercise that will really start to develop and add clarity to those hidden lower abs it's this one! This really is one of my secrets to having such clean cut abdominals so let's make sure we get the technique correct! All we are going to do; is pivot from the hips and bring our knees in towards our chest and then lower them back down to tap the ground. This exercises requires both legs to carry out the same movement together! You will know if you have the correct technique on this exercise; because as you get into the higher repetitions you will feel a really nice burn! (Unsure whether "nice" is the right word here.... oh well.... you decide!)

Beginner: 10 repetitions for 3 sets (30 second break between each set)

Intermediate: 15 repetitions for 3 sets (30 second break between each set)

Advanced: 20 repetitions for 3 sets (30 second break between each set)

Day 3

Side Hip Raises

Good day! I'm glad you have made it to day 3! This is where the fun really begins! Why do i say that? Because you will be happy to know that if you have completed the 5 exercises of day 1 and day 2 you have pretty much covered most areas of the abdominals! However, this is really where we separate the men from the boys and women from the girls! And that's because by now you may have found that you are starting to ache a little and your muscles may be slightly fatigued! This is where it is really important that you are feeding your body the correct things and certainly that you are getting the right amount of protein into your diet as proteins are the building blocks of muscle! No, that does not mean that you are suddenly going to become a bodybuilder by increasing you protein! In fact, increasing your protein is actually a huge factor in increasing your metabolism and therefore assisting you to lose weight! And there you have it; a science lesson in a guide on how to get abs! Of course i go into more detail on this topic in my nutrition guide "The Motivator Meal Plan" but for now; it's time for our Day 3 workout! And to work through the burn!

So, today we are going to begin with Side Hip Raises! We are really going to target those oblique's with this exercise and through consistency with this exercise we will certainly remove those love handles! Make sure that you are nice and stable when carrying out this exercise, we also want to make sure that you aren't putting too much pressure on your back; so ensure that the movement is nice and natural! Let's go!

Beginner: 10 repetitions for 3 sets (30 second break between each set)

Intermediate: 15 repetitions for 3 sets (30 second break between each set)

Advanced: 20 repetitions for 3 sets (30 second break between each set)

Rock and Rollers

No we aren't off to a concert or disco! But we are rocking and rolling towards a Brand New Set of Abs! It's important that we have a little bit of flow and rhythm with this exercise hence the name! What we are going to do is simply crunch up, apply our weight onto out right elbow to help us up, and bring our left elbow to meet our right knee! From this position we will simply roll back down to the starting position before carrying out the exact same action to the other side! Give it try! And remember to have some Rhythm!

Beginner: 10 repetitions for 3 sets (30 second break between each set)

Intermediate: 15 repetitions for 3 sets (30 second break between each set)

Advanced: 20 repetitions for 3 sets (30 second break between each set)

Crunches with legs and chest meeting in the middle

Now! There are a couple of variations to this exercise and on this occasion i have decided to use my arms to demonstrate! However, it is also possible to do this exercise by simply crossing your arms behind your head and following the same instructions! Brilliant, now that you have chosen which variation works best for you and your ability, we are going to simply bring our knees us towards our chest as we also bring our chest forward (meet in the middle). Once, you have done this, lower both your legs and torso back down and that is one repetition complete! Let's work!

Beginner: 10 repetitions for 3 sets (30 second break between each set)

Intermediate: 15 repetitions for 3 sets (30 second break between each set)

Advanced: 20 repetitions for 3 sets (30 second break between each set)

Mountain Climbers

It's time for mountain climbers! And to work those lower abs whilst also working on achieving that perfect V-Shape! Notice that we have previously worked the oblique's during our "Drunken Mountain Climber" activity on day 1! This time we are totally sober! (I hope) as we are going to be doing straight Mountain Clumbers. From the neutral (high lank) position, we are simply going to bring one leg into our chest and then back down into the neutral position. Once we have done this; we will then bring the opposite leg up and back down into the neutral position. You guessed correctly! Once you have completed both legs; this is 1 repetition!

Beginner: 30 second burst of exercise for 3 sets (follow each set with a 30 second break)

Intermediate: 45 second burst of exercise for 3 sets (follow each set with a 30 second break)

Advanced: 1 minute burst of exercise for 3 sets (follow each set with a 30 second break)

Scissor Kicks

We are now onto our final exercise for day 3! If you have followed each activity correctly; after this final exercise of the day you can give yourself a BIG pat on the back as we have come a very long way to developing those perfect abs! We are going to finish today with Scissor Kicks! Scissor Kicks are a fantastic way to work those abs and also increase your core strength and stability! Let's get those super flat stomachs! All we are going to do; is lie flat in a neutral position with our arms out to the side...(There is a method of making this exercise slightly easier by placing our hands underneath our bottom's!). Once your hands are in position, keep your neck nice and straight and raise your right leg into the air (keeping it nice and straight) once you have reached a 45 degree angle, lower your right leg down to 1inch from the ground (do not touch the floor) and now do the same with the left leg! It's very important that we do not rush this exercise, it's not a race! So we want to make sure that this is a nice steady and controlled movement! It's Scissor Time!

Beginner: 10 repetitions for 3 sets (30 second break between each set)

Intermediate: 15 repetitions for 3 sets (30 second break between each set)

Advanced: 20 repetitions for 3 sets (30 second break between each set)

Day 4

The Plank

I feel your pain! But it's time to Kick Start Day 4! Believe me, I know exactly how you feel. Just one more day tomorrow and then we can rest these abdominals and follow "The Motivator Meal Guide" to help repair and rebuild these abdominals! At least we are going to begin day 4 by remaining nice and still with The Plank! That's fair? Right, so with this exercise it's very important that we keep our abdominals engaged throughout. The reason I mention this, is because if we have our bottoms too high up we disengage the abs and also if we have our torso too low we will disengage the abs. Hence the name "The Plank" We want to keep our cores nice and tight and really feel the squeeze in this region! This honestly is such a fantastic exercise for strengthening and defining our middles!

Beginner: 30 second burst of exercise for 3 sets (follow each set with a 30 second break)

Intermediate: 45 second burst of exercise for 3 sets (follow each set with a 30 second break)

Advanced: 1 minute burst of exercise for 3 sets (follow each set with a 30 second break)

Lower Abs

Can you remember our reverse crunch exercise? The one that was one of my favourite exercises for defining those lower abs? Well let's call this exercise The Big Brother! It's very similar that we are simply going to bring our knees up towards our stomach. However, this time around it's going to be 1 knee at a time! From the neutral position (with your arms out to the side) bring one leg up to your stomach and then back down so that the toe of this leg literally "taps" the floor. Once back into the neutral position; it's now time to go again with the opposite leg. As with all the Motivator Exercises; once you have completed the exercise with both legs; that will be 1 repetition!

Beginner: 10 repetitions for 3 sets (30 second break between each set)

Intermediate: 15 repetitions for 3 sets (30 second break between each set)

Advanced: 20 repetitions for 3 sets (30 second break between each set)

Criss-cross Legs

I didn't want to give too much away with the name; but i suppose it just couldn't be described any other way! This exercise is extremely similar to the Scissor Kicks Exercise we touched on at the final exercise of Day 3! But, this time; rather than raising our legs directly up and down, we are literally going to be "Criss-Crossing" our legs in the middle of the air. Yes, that's right over left and then left over right for one repetition! As with the Scissor Kicks, It's very important to remember that this exercise should be carried out in a nice controlled manor!

Beginner: 10 repetitions for 3 sets (30 second break between each set)

Intermediate: 15 repetitions for 3 sets (30 second break between each set)

Advanced: 20 repetitions for 3 sets (30 second break between each set)

Long Arm Crunches

Now, let's work the muscles towards the top of our abdominals! This exercise is very similar to a crunch. However, instead of the conventional crunch; in this exercise we are going to stretch our arms out nice and long in the neutral position! Now, as we come up towards our knees, we have isolated the abs as we cannot swing our arms or use the momentum to bring us up! This is a great exercise and also stops any cheating from occurring! If you get the technique right with this one; you will certainly feel those abs working! 3, 2, 1 Go!

Beginner: 10 repetitions for 3 sets (30 second break between each set)

Intermediate: 15 repetitions for 3 sets (30 second break between each set)

Advanced: 20 repetitions for 3 sets (30 second break between each set)

V -sit Knee Raises

So we have arrived at the final exercise of day 4! We have battled our way through and we can almost stand victorious that we have completed 4 full days of The Motivator Guide to Abs! But don't celebrate too soon, many have tried and failed at this hurdle... But not you! Today i believe you can overcome the V-Sit Knee Raises and continue on to your final workout of the week tomorrow! Sitting in the V Position is going to really ensure that your abs are consistently working throughout this exercise! Once in position, simply bring your knees into your chest nice and controlled; and then lower them back down until you are just 1inch from the floor. You will be bringing both knees into your chest at the same time when carrying out this exercise; meaning once you bought them into your chest and back down that is 1 repetition! You can do it!

Beginner: 10 repetitions for 3 sets (30 second break between each set)

Intermediate: 15 repetitions for 3 sets (30 second break between each set)

Advanced: 20 repetitions for 3 sets (30 second break between each set)

Day 5

Sitting Twists

I'm so excited for today's workout! Not only does it mean you have completed 5 full days of my guide to those perfect abs; but after today you have also earned 2 well deserved rest days to give our muscles a chance to grow! Today we are going to begin with Sitting Twists also known as Russian Twists! They are an incredible way to increase your core strength, reduce fats and also build better stability! It's Go time!

Beginner: 10 repetitions for 3 sets (30 second break between each set)

Intermediate: 15 repetitions for 3 sets (30 second break between each set)

Advanced: 20 repetitions for 3 sets (30 second break between each set)

Push Up To Plank

Now, now, now! Push up to plank is a great test of both core and arm strength! Don't worry it sounds a lot more complicated than it actually is and you won't be doing full push ups during this exercise! First of all you will need to begin in the raised plan position with your arms nice and straight. From this position you are simply going to come down onto either elbow to begin with and then follow by also going onto the elbow of your other arm. Now you should be on both elbows! (Plank Position). From this position, simply get back up into the starting position by firstly straightening one arm (preferably the first arm you lead the exercise with) and the second arm! You will be happy to know that is one repetition! How many can you complete during the times specified below:

Beginner: 30 second burst of exercise for 3 sets (follow each set with a 30 second break)

Intermediate: 45 second burst of exercise for 3 sets (follow each set with a 30 second break)

Advanced: 1 minute burst of exercise for 3 sets (follow each set with a 30 second break)

Crunches hands over knees

It's time for a more direct abdominal exercise! With this exercise you will begin in a neutral position with your knees bent, back straight and arms resting on your thighs. From this position; you are simply going to engage your abs, reach up and touch just over the top of your knees, before returning back to the neutral position! During this exercise as with all other abdominal exercises, it is important not to put too much pressure on your neck by changing positions suddenly. Try to maintain a nice straight posture, with your chest out wherever you possibly can.

Beginner: 10 repetitions for 3 sets (30 second break between each set)

Intermediate: 15 repetitions for 3 sets (30 second break between each set)

Advanced: 20 repetitions for 3 sets (30 second break between each set)

6 inches

Anybody who has trained in boxing for any period of time will definitely be familiar with the famous 6 inches! For this exercise i would like you to begin by lying flat in a neutral position with your arms out to the side (once again you can place your hands under your bottom if you would like to make this slightly easier). From this position, whilst your back and neck is nice and flat; I would like you to raise both of your legs at the same time; just 6 inches off the ground. Of course i don't require you to get a measuring tape out; but if you are unsure of how high 6 inches is (approximately) you may want to remind yourself! Right! Once, you are in this position, it's time to simply sit still and enjoy that feeling! Let's hold the 6 inches for the amount of time specified below before returning to the neutral position with your feet on the floor for a 30 seconds break.

Beginner: 30 second burst of exercise for 3 sets (follow each set with a 30 second break)

Intermediate: 45 second burst of exercise for 3 sets (follow each set with a 30 second break)

Advanced: 1 minute burst of exercise for 3 sets (follow each set with a 30 second break)

High Knees on the Spot

You have made it! Congratulations on making it this far! You have now reached your final ab exercise of the week and you should be feeling extremely proud! You will also be happy to know that this one is a nice and easy way to finish and to shake off those cobwebs! We are going to finish with some nice high knees on the spot! High knees are a fantastic way to engage your abs when carried out correctly! One leg at a time we are simply going to raise our knee and along with the opposite arm and alternate for the amount of time specified below based on your ability. Remember once again that this is not a race (although it will look like you are running) but more about engaging those abs. Keep your core nice and tight and keep both good balance and control.

Beginner: 30 second burst of exercise for 3 sets (follow each set with a 30 second break)

Intermediate: 45 second burst of exercise for 3 sets (follow each set with a 30 second break)

Advanced: 1 minute burst of exercise for 3 sets (follow each set with a 30 second break)

What happens next?

You've Made it this far and you are now about to unwind for 2 full days of rest. (Rest is advised for specifically the abs, of course if you continue to workout during these 2 days, just ensure you are primarily working other muscle groups). I would also advise checking out "The Motivator Meal Plan" during this time; as by getting the right nutrients and amounts of protein into the body during this period is vital to optimum repair.

Now that you have completed the first 5 days and are about to go into your rest period. I thought it would be a nice time to tell you that over the next 3 weeks we are going to continue wand be consistent with our workout plan of 5 days' work and 2 days' rest. Simply using the 5 day workout guide above; we will continue this regime for a total of 4 weeks (3 weeks remaining). At this point I would advise carrying out your activities on the same days each week; this will allow for you to have sufficient workout and rest periods.

Your 4 Week Structure

So here we have it! Your 4 week structure!

Week 1 – Day 1 workout, Day 2 workout, Day 3 workout, Day 4 workout, Day 5 workout, Rest Day, Rest Day.

Week 2 - Day 1 workout, Day 2 workout, Day 3 workout, Day 4 workout, Day 5 workout, Rest Day, Rest Day

Week 3 - Day 1 workout, Day 2 workout, Day 3 workout, Day 4 workout, Day 5 workout, Rest

Day, Rest Day

Week 4 - Day 1 workout, Day 2 workout, Day 3 workout, Day 4 workout, Day 5 workout, Rest Day, Rest Day

Important Facts from Kurt Motivator

Kurt Motivator Suggests having an easily digestible protein/carbohydrate source within the 30 minute window following your daily ab workout.

Remember that a large part of abdominal definition is down to your nutrition and diet, this guide used in combination with the 80% (nutrition) will take your abs to a whole new level of definition.

This guide is aimed to hit your abs from a variety of different movements and techniques. In Kurt's opinion; if you follow this guide correctly and complete each exercise for the recommended time period, the no additional abdominal exercises should be required during the 4 week period.

Of course, once you have completed the 4 week guide combined with good nutrition; and have seen the changes take place before your eyes. The fun doesn't have to stop there! Kurt suggests integrating the 4 week guide and structure repeatedly for enhanced results. Variety is the key and this workout certainly contains variety that hit your muscles from many different angles.

It is very important to remain hydrated. It's a known fact that drinking water can actually assist with losing weight by helping to flush many of those bad toxins we don't want in our bodies out of our system! You will be surprised how increasing your water intake can contribute and speed up the process of achieving those clean abs!

Has the Motivator Guide to abs worked for you?

If, like so many others around the UK and internationally you have found that The Motivator Guide to abs has assisted you in achieving the results you desired. Why not refer this guide to two friends and receive 20% discount off The Motivator Meal Plan. Here is the process:

Direct two friends to kurtmotivator.bigcartel.com who would like to order "The Motivator Guide to Abs" > Once they have ordered, YOUR full name and address along with their names to kurtisshinner@live.co.uk and we will respond with your 20% discount.

Alternatively, you can head over to the Official Facebook Page – Kurt Motivator Official and share "The Motivator Guide to Abs" post to be in with a chance of winning a FREE copy of The Motivator Meal Plan.

"I sincerely hope that this guide has given you huge value and a better understanding, but most of all a better physique! Smaller love handles! And Even More Confidence!"

Best Wishes,

Kurt Motivator

E: kurtisshinner@live.co.uk

F: Kurt Motivator Official

Need more assistance with form? Here is Your Image Guide:

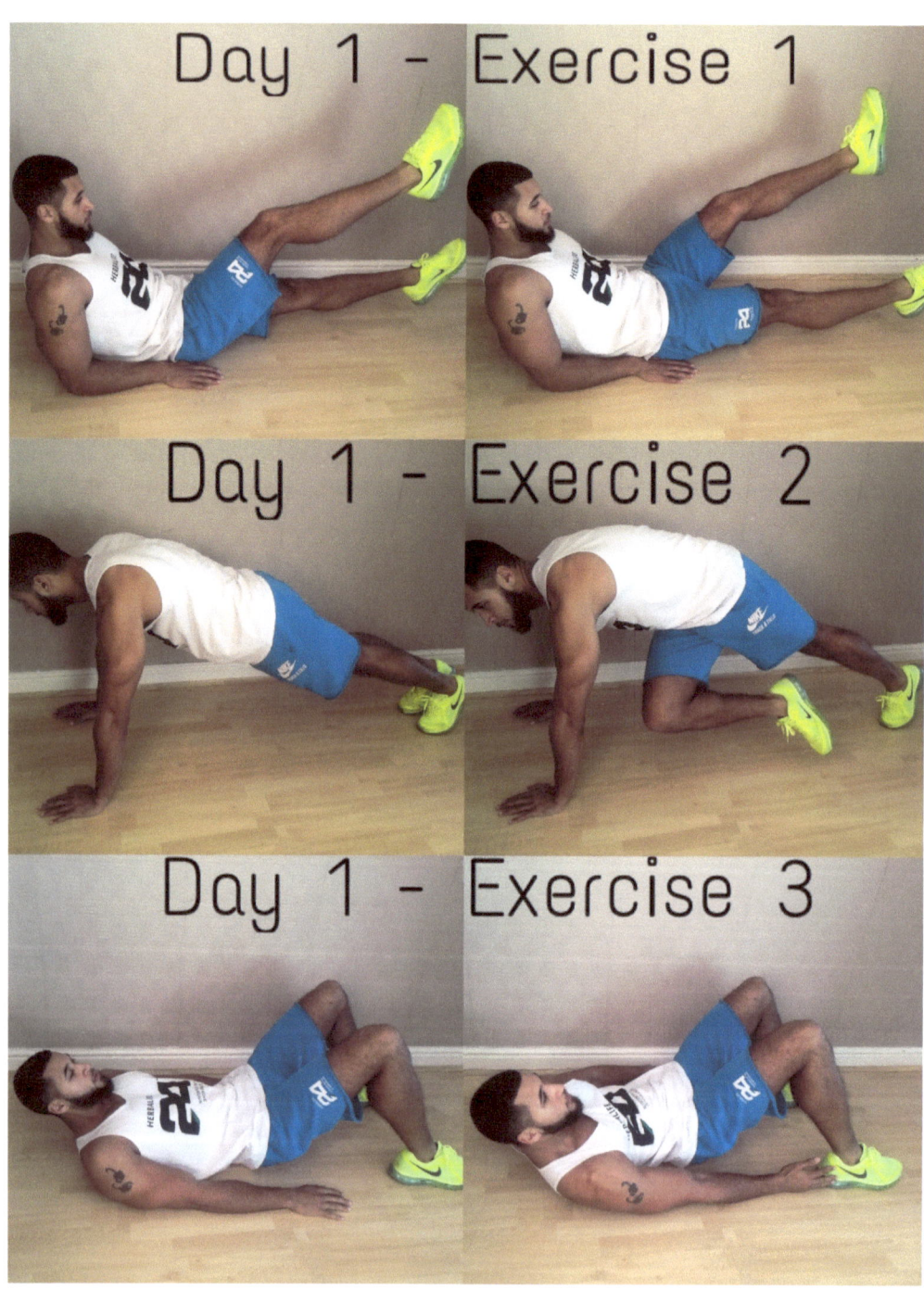

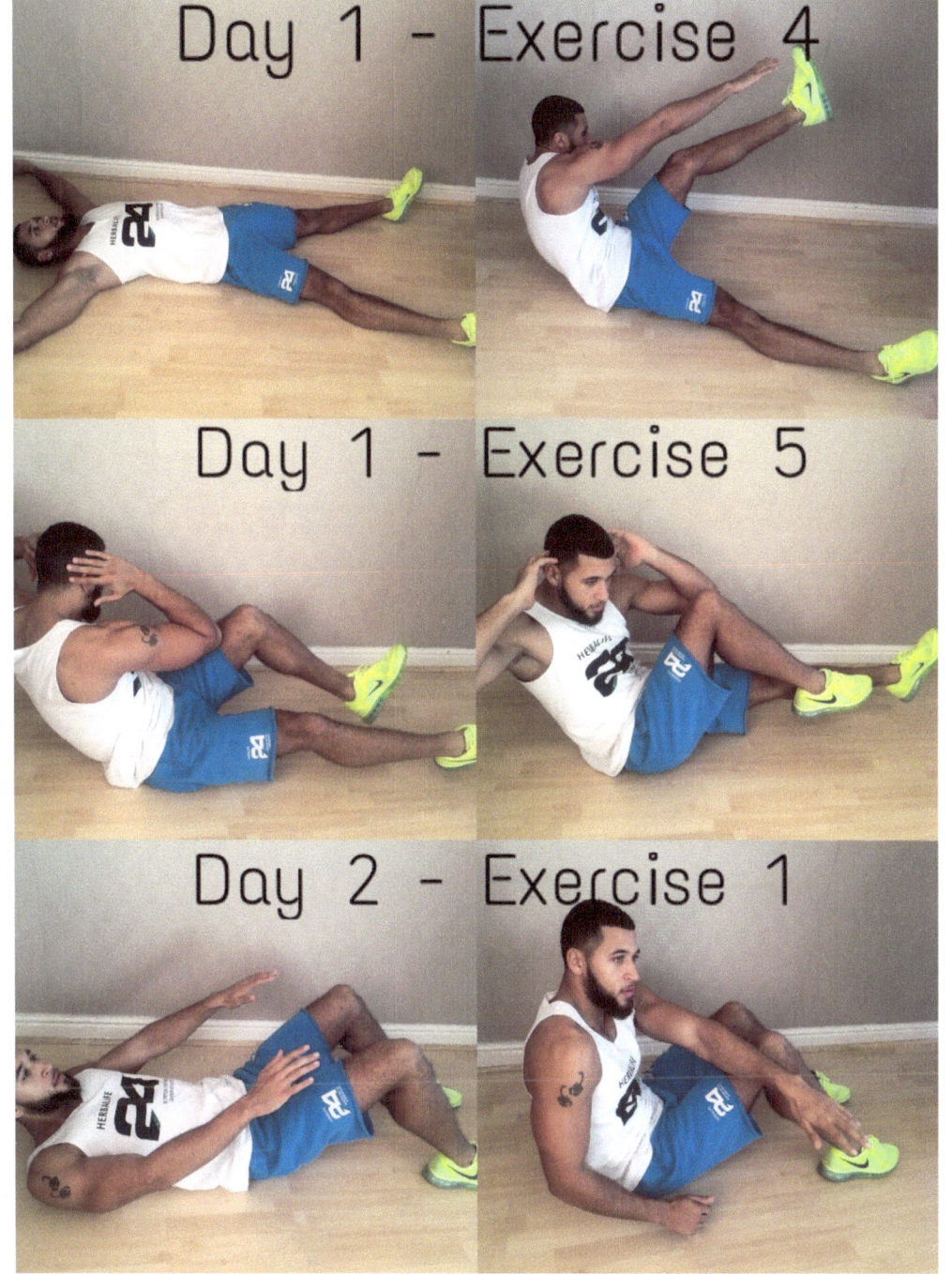

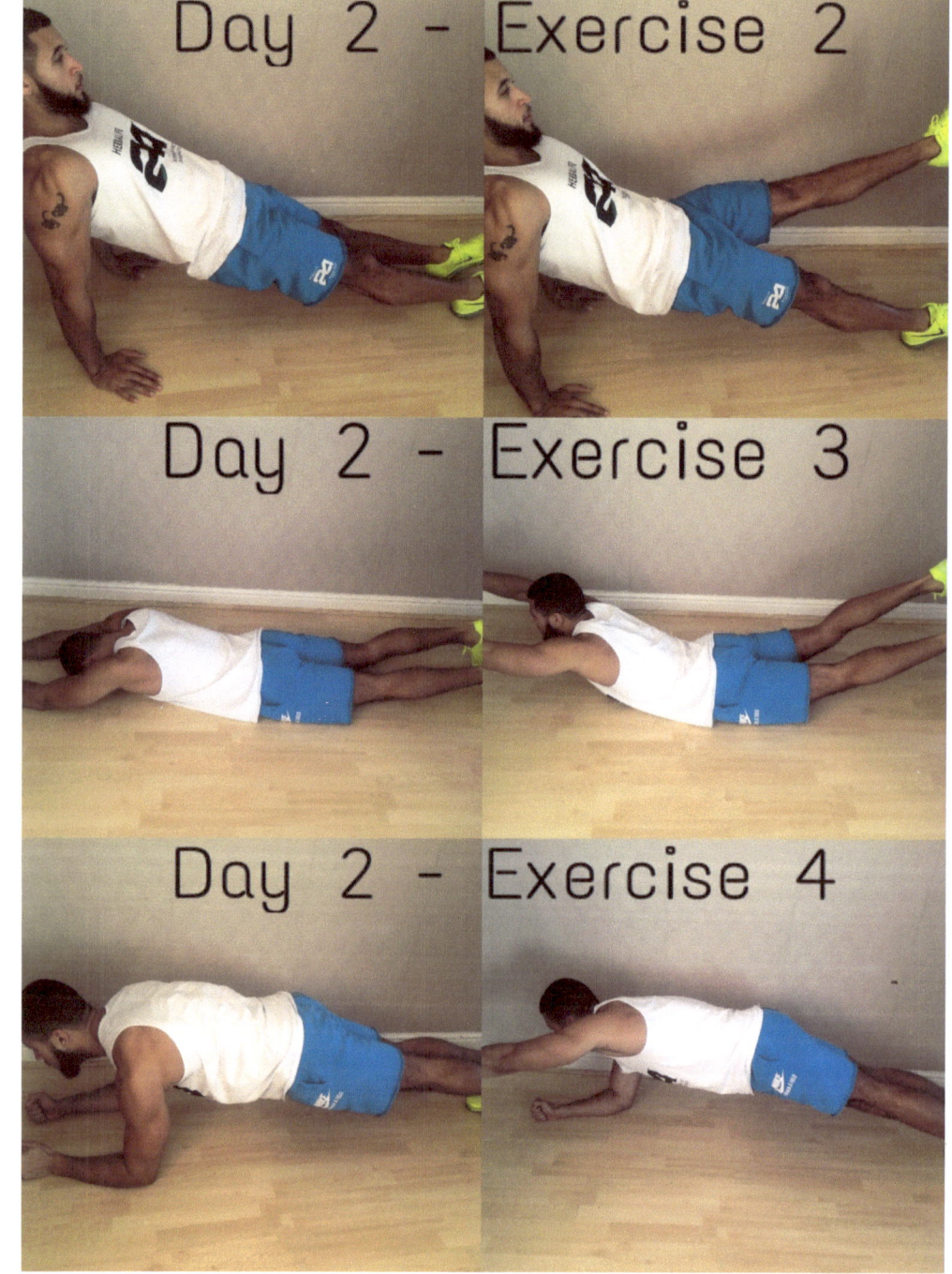

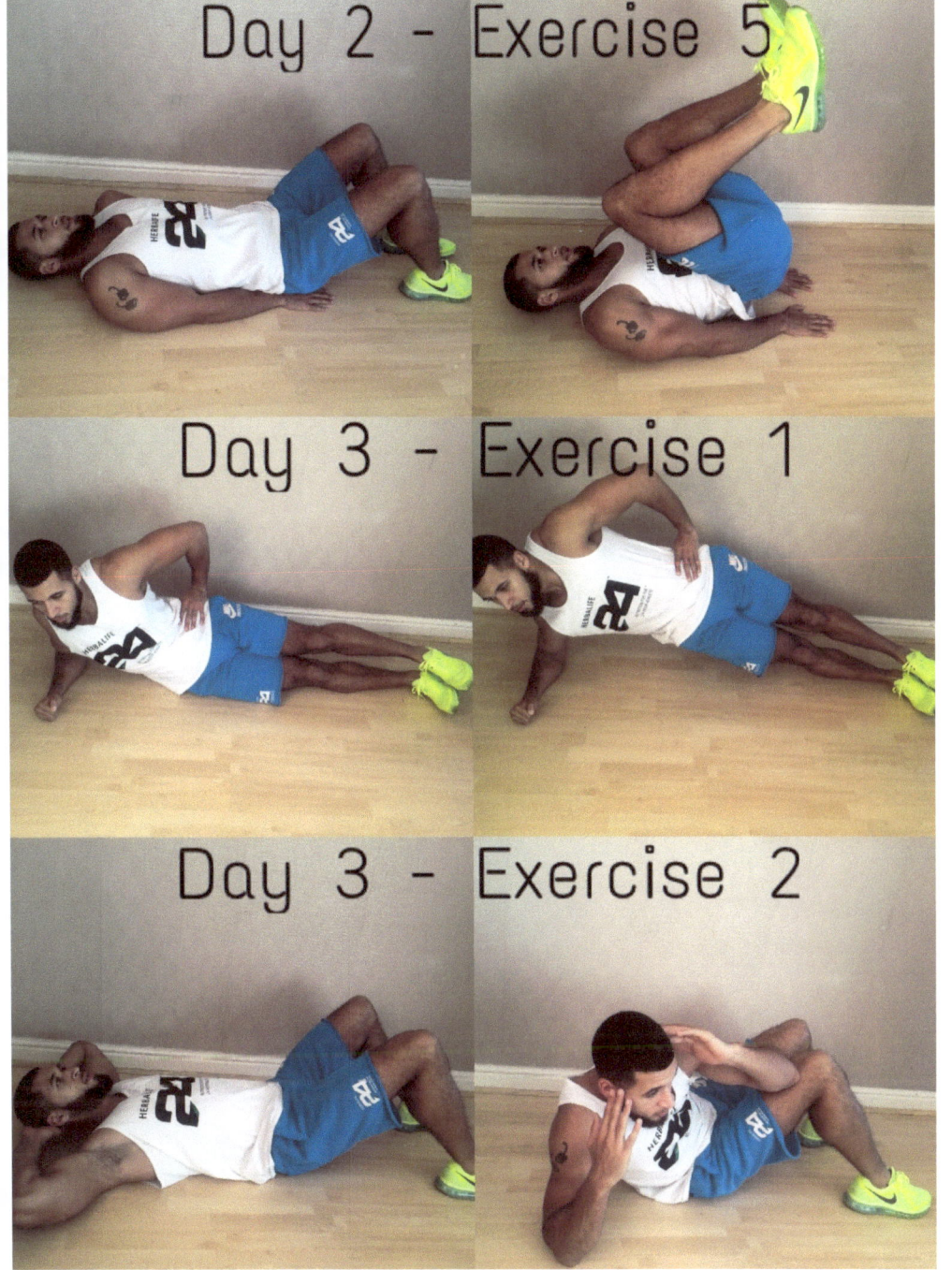

Day 2 - Exercise 5

Day 3 - Exercise 1

Day 3 - Exercise 2

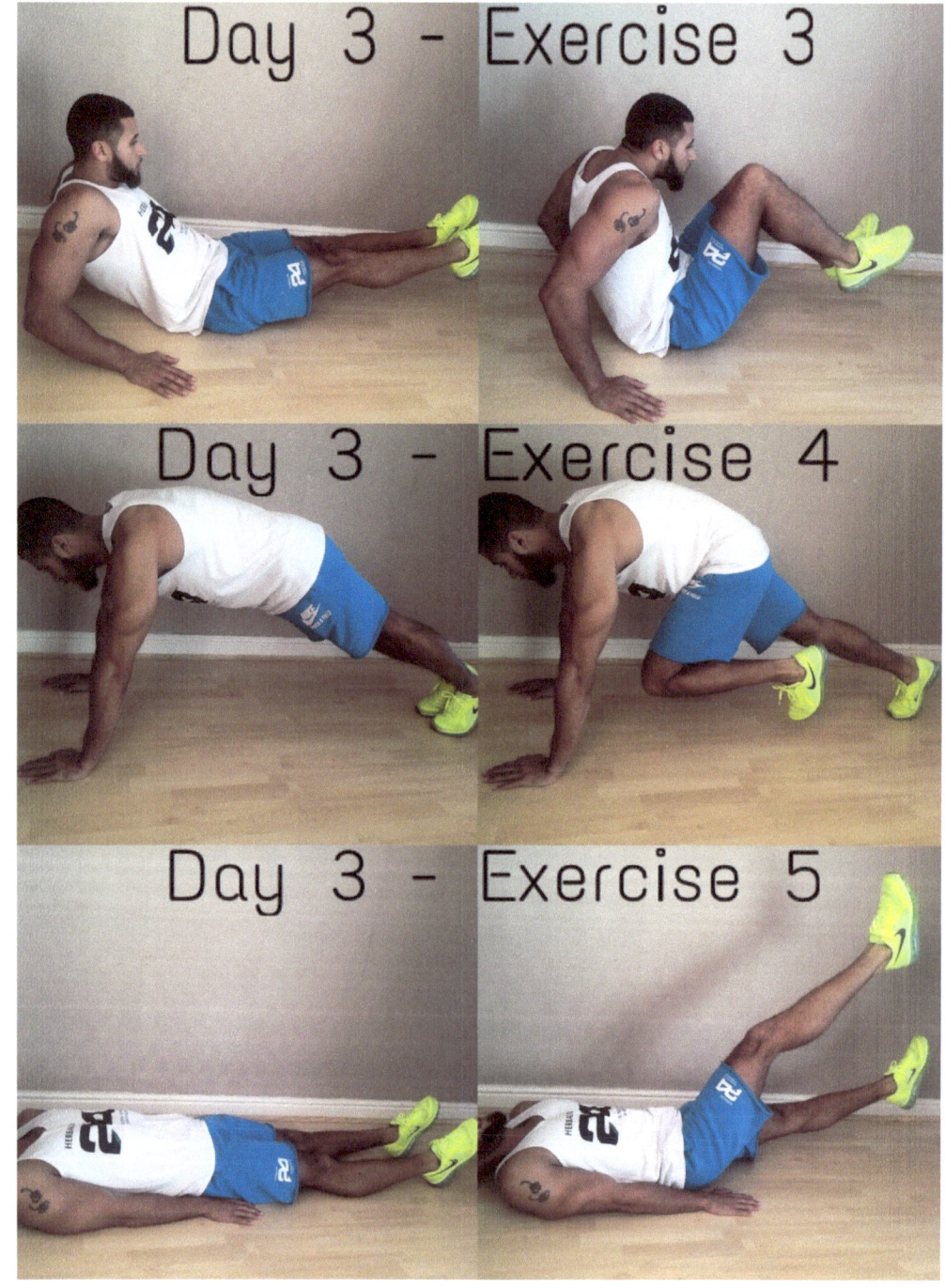

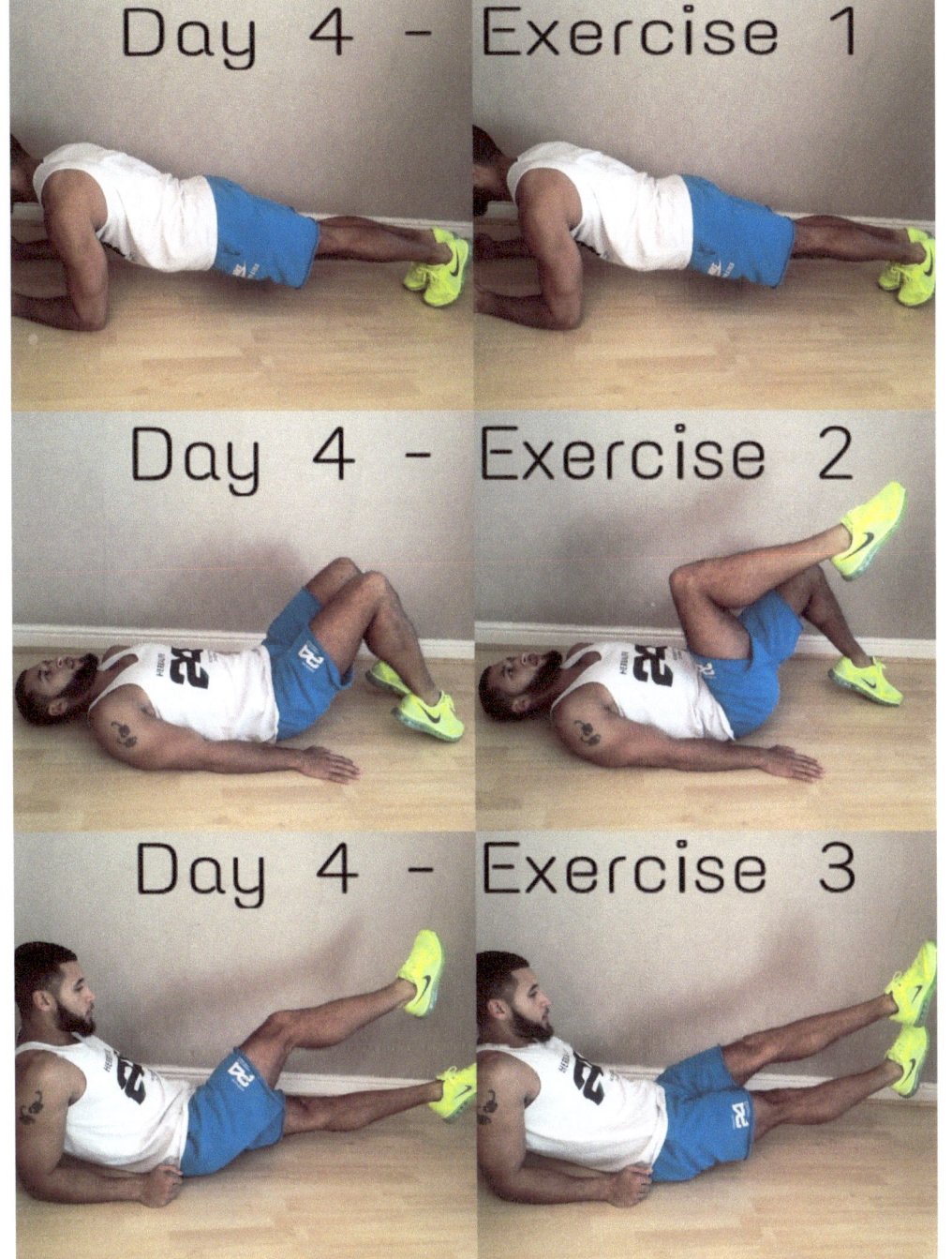

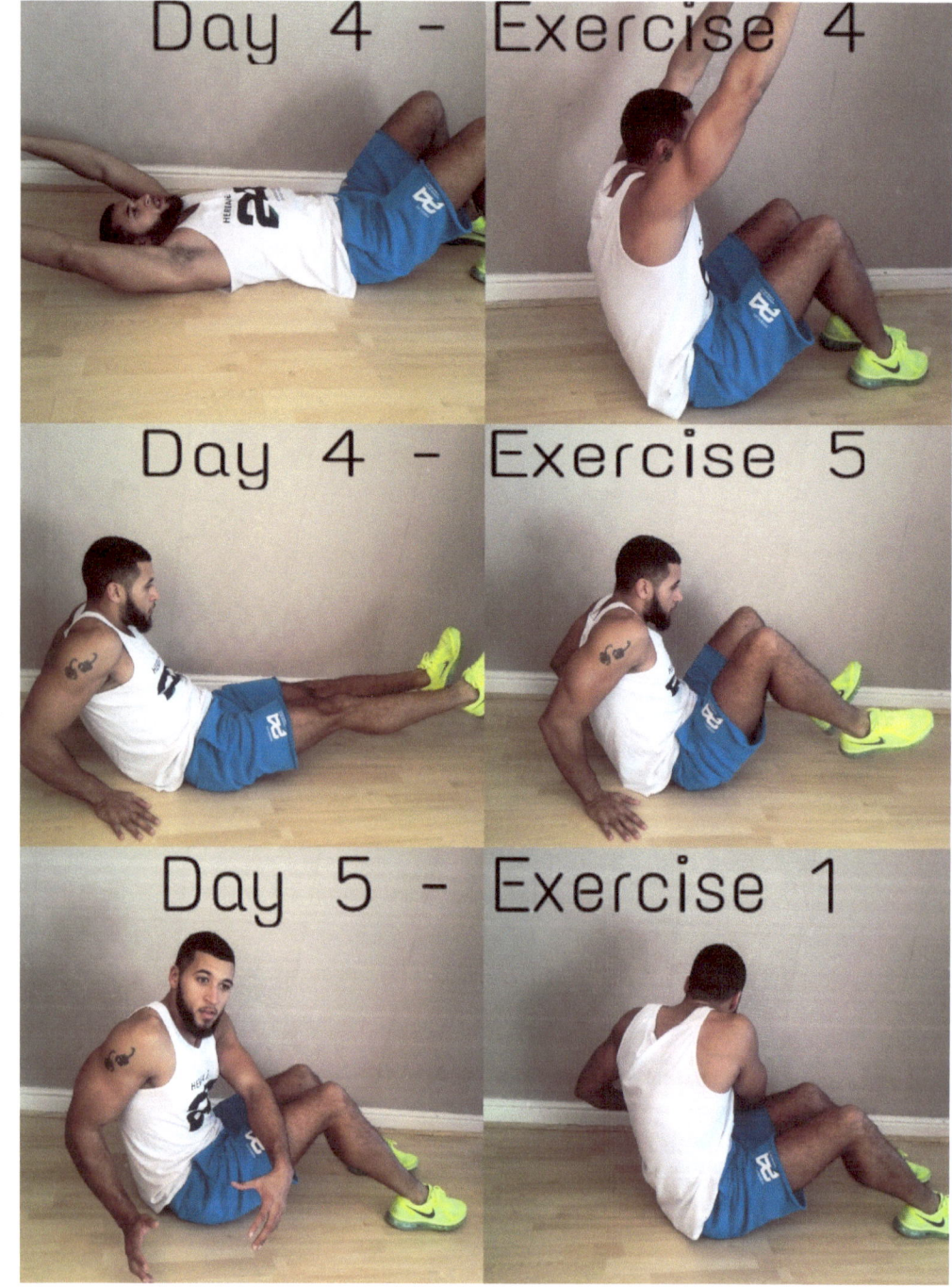

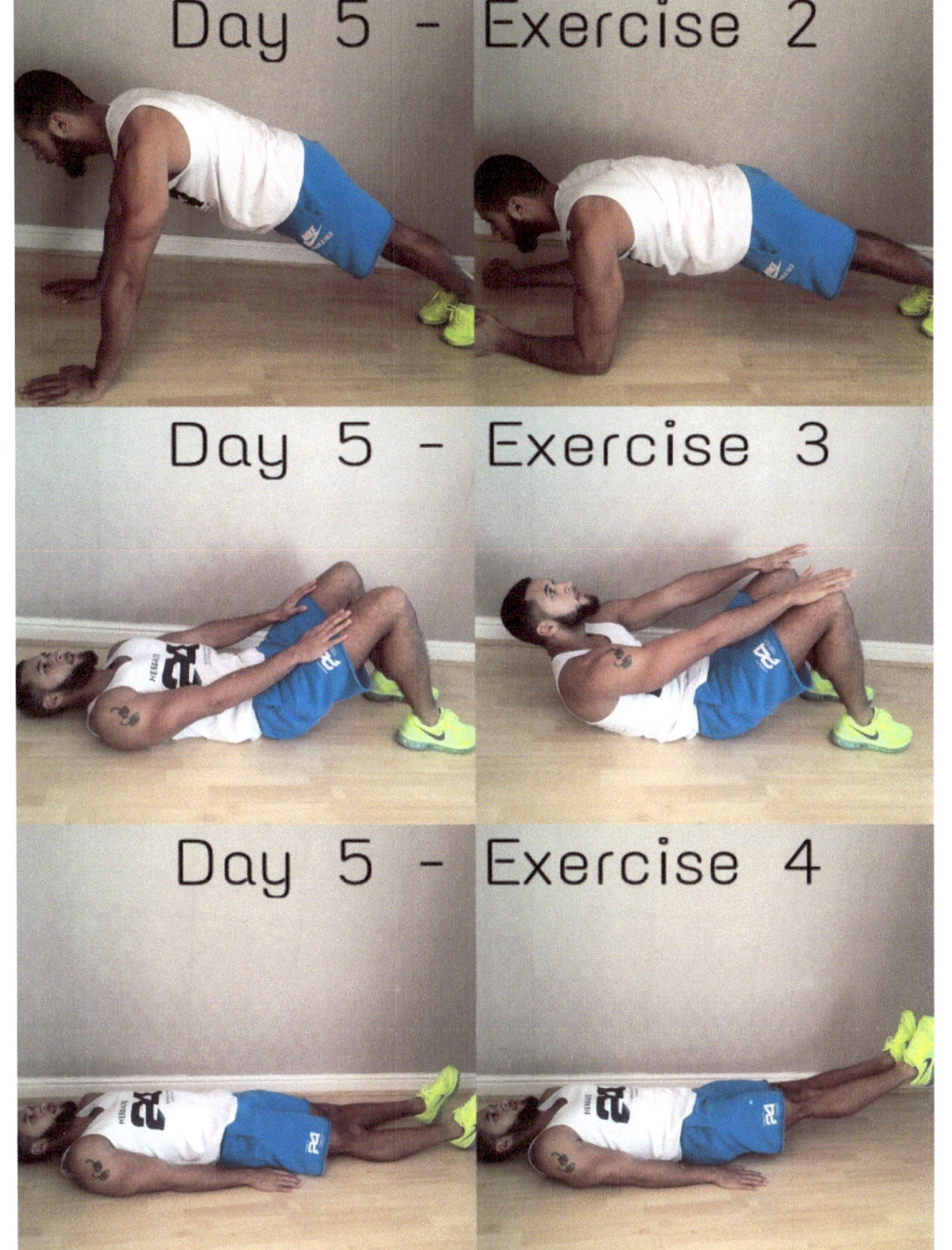

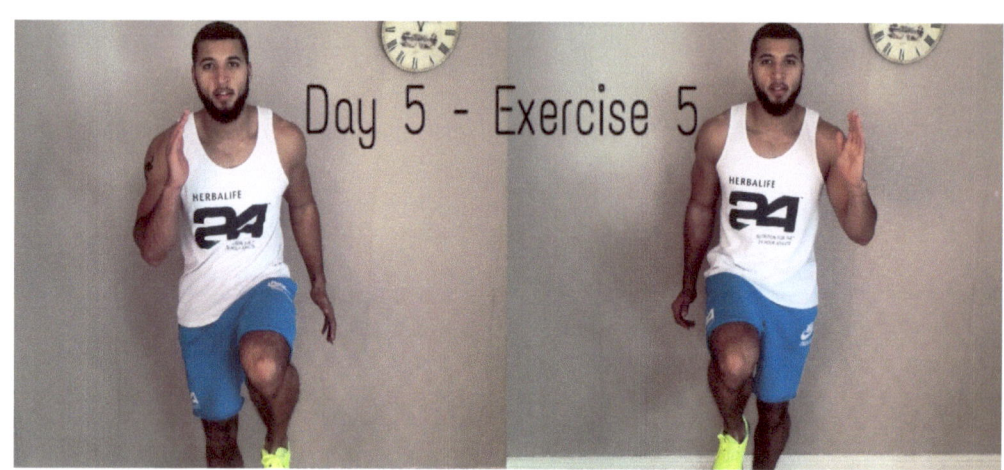

Day 5 - Exercise 5

www.ingramcontent.com/pod-product-compliance
Lightning Source LLC
Chambersburg PA
CBHW050933290526
45792CB00002B/998